CANCER

A TRUE STORY OF COURAGE, HOPE AND SURVIVAL

ELSIE YOUNG

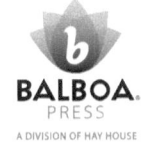

BALBOA
PRESS

A DIVISION OF HAY HOUSE

Balboa Press books may be ordered through booksellers or by contacting:

Balboa Press
A Division of Hay House
1663 Liberty Drive
Bloomington, IN 47403
www.balboapress.com
1 (877) 407-4847

Print information available on the last page.

ISBN: 978-1-5043-9432-1 (sc)
ISBN: 978-1-5043-9493-2 (hc)
ISBN: 978-1-5043-9433-8 (e)

Balboa Press rev. date: 02/07/2018

I dedicate this book to my children: Anthony, Angela, Adria, and Alex. For your love, kindness, and devotion, and for your endless support.

CONTENTS

Preface xi

Chapter 1   The Shocking News 1
Chapter 2   A Diagnosis Is Made 9
Chapter 3   My New Oncologist 19
Chapter 4   My Treatment Plan 23
Chapter 5   Medication-Induced Acute Hepatitis B: Liver
            Failure 33
Chapter 6   Very Dramatic 41
Chapter 7   Despondent Yet Elated 49
Chapter 8   A Great New Beginning 57
Chapter 9   Tips and Ideas 61

Epilogue 65
Acknowledgments 67
Inspirational Notes 75

I draw this for my mother to use in her book. Alex Young.
Email permission.
Mr. Toby

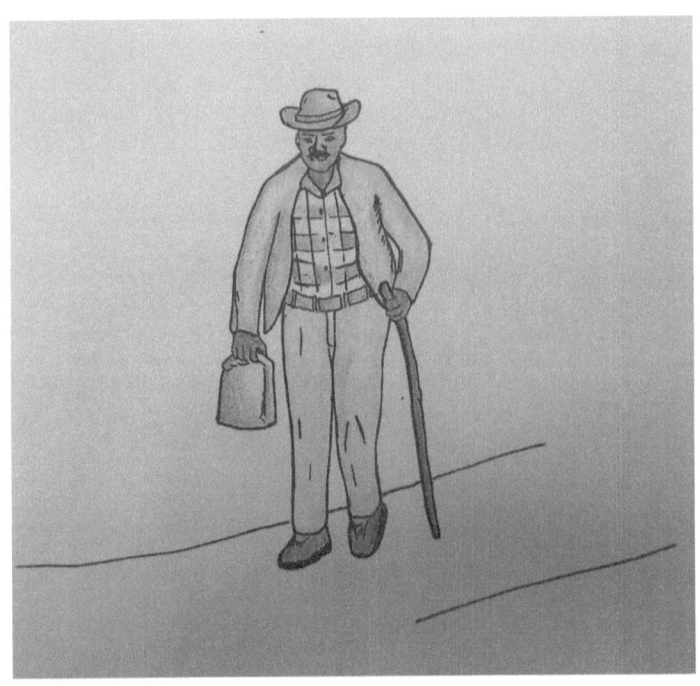

PREFACE

It is my desire that this book will provide genuine hope, wisdom, and optimism to those who are struggling with their cancer journeys. In this book, you'll read my thoughts, discover my strength, and marvel at the many obstacles I had with doctors on my cancer journey. Their names are changed to protect their identities. I tried to be as accurate as possible so that readers can hear the voice of my experiences. I hope you'll laugh reading this, as well as occasionally wipe some tears from your eyes. It's a sad story at times, but there is also much to learn here. Please, sit back, relax, and enjoy the read.

PREFACE

THE SHOCKING NEWS

I was at the hospital, unconscious from the anesthesia and waiting for the physician to remove the shunt he had inserted, when I saw myself lying on a bed on a runway. It was an airstrip in a field, with bushes all around and no buildings in sight. The runway looked brand new, like it was just paved and had never been used. Deep yellow lines in the center looked freshly painted. I lay on a bed at one end of the runway. At the other end was a private jet. Suddenly, I heard footsteps running toward me, but I saw no one. The footsteps were running very fast, coming at me, and then I heard a voice: "Is this my patient?" the voice said. "Move away, move away." I recalled this weeks after my procedure but never mentioned it to anyone.

It had all started five years earlier, on a beautiful September evening in 2011. I was excited to be meeting with a new patient; I was a caregiver, a certified nurse's assistant. As I was getting dressed, I felt something running down my face and realized I was having a nosebleed. In all of my fifty-plus years, I'd never had a nosebleed. I was never sick; I'd had no illnesses besides childhood measles and colds here and there. Quickly, I took a piece of tissue and tried to stop the bleeding, but it was useless. The blood was thick, and no intervention to stop the bleeding seemed to work. The nosebleed lasted for about one hour. Considering that I'd never been sick before this nosebleed, I was frightened. I saw health insurance as an unnecessary expense, and therefore didn't have any. The only health issue I experienced was fatigue: I would go to sleep tired and wake up tired, but I never considered that a big deal. I thought it was just part of getting older. Once the nosebleed stopped, I never thought about it again.

My father was an herbalist. When I was young, many people knew him as the medicine man because of his knowledge of healing plants, the knowledge that was handed down to him from his father. It amazed me that these men knew so much and had no formal education. As a child, I was always by my father's side when he cultivated these plants, which were planted on the hill just behind our farmhouse. He grew all the vegetables, herbs, and flowers for his home remedies from seeds. Ingredients he used for his medicines could include honey, onions, garlic, tree bark, and animal fat. He completely cured one of my sisters of asthma with his medicines. My father noticed my interest in his medicines and would often say to me, "You should be a nurse." But I couldn't imagine being a nurse and taking care of sick people. Instead, I grew up to work in several different fields. First, I worked at a radio station, summarizing stories for children. After that, I worked in the banking field for many years, in the accounting and funds management departments. My passion, however, lies in creative arts, and I went on to become an entrepreneurial garden designer, creating garden designs for private clients to enhance their home environment.

One day, to my surprise, a very close friend in the medical field asked me to help her with one of her patients. Right away I told her that was something I could not do. The patient, my friend, said, needed help and did not have serious health conditions. She was a senior and primarily needed care and companionship. "Elsie," she said, "you can do it. It's like taking care of a baby." Well, I knew how to do that, since I had raised my children and helped my sisters with theirs; I agreed to help.

My friend went away for a couple of days, and I took care of the patient, thinking of her as my child and giving her the care and companionship she needed. I could tell she was very appreciative and happy with how I was caring for her. When my friend moved away a few weeks later, I was offered the opportunity to be one of the patient's caregivers. When this wonderful lady died seven months later, I decided to enroll in classes and become a certified nurse's assistant (CNA). I loved what I was doing as a CNA and started taking classes to become a licensed practical nurse.

I was in my fifties when I embarked on this positive and refreshing new career as a healthcare provider, doing in-home care. I liked it so much that I wondered why I hadn't gotten into the medical field earlier, as my father had suggested. I know he would be pleased with what I am doing, just as he must have been happy to give the care that is so desperately needed. A year and a half later, I was offered a job as a caregiver for a ninety-seven-year-old gentleman in Pennsylvania. The gentleman sounded like a very interesting person, so I took the job and made a move from Florida to Pennsylvania.

One evening, just as I was about to start preparing dinner, the second episode of my nosebleeds started. This time, fortunately, the episode was not as severe—just a small drop of blood and it was over. I assured myself this had happened because of the cold winter weather. The dripping ended up going on for about ten days.

As a caregiver, I now had health insurance through my employer, so I decided to see a doctor about the bleeding. I made an appointment with my primary care physician, Dr. Mack, and also made an appointment with Dr. Uribe, an ear, nose, and throat specialist (ENT). At the examination, Dr. Mack told me the problem was hypertension—high blood pressure. Medication for it would stop my nosebleeds, he said. I started taking the prescribed medication for hypertension immediately, and sure enough, my nosebleeds stopped. I canceled the ENT appointment.

About three weeks later, the nosebleeds were back, and this time they were much more severe. I went to see Dr. Uribe, the ENT specialist, who cauterized the inside of both nostrils. This seals the blood vessels that builds scar tissue, to help prevent more bleeding. This helped for a few days, and then the bleeding started again. I was at that office two or three times a week seeing Dr. Uribe or one of the other ENTs. I became fearful they might think I had Munchausen syndrome, a mental disorder in which a person repeatedly injures themselves to seek attention or sympathy, but these doctors showed me only compassion.

Meanwhile, the nosebleeds continued, without warning. I was at a restaurant one day, having lunch with a friend, when a gush of blood started pouring down my face. I had to leave in a hurry. After that, I was paralyzed with fear, afraid to do anything or go anywhere. I was a nervous wreck. What in the world was happening to me? I used to be a strong, healthy person. Was this what aging was all about: things just creep up out of nowhere? The bleeding continued for months.

I decided to go back to see Dr. Mack, my primary care physician, who gave me a prescription for lab work. A few days later I stopped by his office to inquire about the result. This was a very small town, and appointments to see the doctor weren't always needed. Dr. Mack rustled through some papers to find mine, looked them over, and then said something I would come to learn was quite significant: "There is too much protein in your blood," he told me.

"Oh?" I said. "Do I need to cut back on the amount of protein I'm eating?"

"No," he said. "Let's do some more lab work." More tests followed, and when the results of those tests came back, Dr. Mack told me my body was making a different type of protein. "Not good!" he said.

"What is the name of this bad protein my body is making?" I asked.

"It could be cancer." He said those words in a serious tone. "But I am not sure."

I felt like I was punched in the gut. Cancer had never crossed my mind even once.

"Cancer!" I shouted. "How can that be?"

He saw how shocked and frightened I was, and trying to calm me down, he said, "I am not sure it is cancer. Therefore a bone marrow biopsy will have to be done."

"What's the cost of that?" I asked.

"I don't know the cost of procedures or medications," said Dr. Mack, "so I don't make decisions about who can or cannot afford the treatments needed." He referred me to a hematologist, Dr. Ramer, saying that he would send my lab results there to get his opinion. "Not to worry," he told me. "If it is cancer, it is slow growing. You are not feeling sick beside the nosebleeds, and you haven't lost any weight."

It was August 2013, and the insurance company would not pay for any procedures needed because this was considered a pre-existing condition. Dr. Mack advised me to wait until the next year to proceed, when the Affordable Care Act (ACA) kicked in. I left the doctor's office stunned. I sat in my car in complete despair, paralyzed with fear, wondering how this could be happening to me. I always ate healthy, and I was never sick. I felt alone, so very alone. I have never felt such deep loneliness. I drove off, knowing that I couldn't tell anyone about this.

At home, I went to my room and fell on my knees. I cried out to God.

"Lord," I prayed, "I put this in your hands. Please heal my body from whatever is going on." Tears, not blood, were streaming down my face. I buried my face in my pillow and cried for what felt like hours. After my prayer, I got up from my knees, feeling refreshed. It felt like a new dawn with fresh dew on the grass, like a ray of sunshine with a rainbow in the sky after a storm. A load had been lifted, and I knew I could go on because I was no longer alone. I reached out to my home church, telling them about my nosebleeds and asking for prayers. Words cannot express my deep gratitude for them. I have never felt such deep loneliness again.

About two weeks later, I went to see the hematologist, Dr. Ramer. His office was empty, except for maybe one other patient. (I love these small towns!) I gave the staff my information and was put into a room. In less than five minutes, Dr. Ramer came in. He was a small man, looking to be in his mid-fifties, with a brown complexion showing the features of Indian decent. He didn't sit in a chair; he leaned against the wall and slid down to a squatting position. I laughed to myself.

"Hello," he said, speaking with a distinct Indian accent. "And why are you here?" I was a little taken aback by his question."

Haven't you received my lab results from my primary care physician, Dr. Mack?"

"Oh, just a minute." He went out and returned with a folder, and then he went back to his squatting position near the wall and flipped through the papers. "Your protein is very high." He called for his nurse. "Set up for a bone marrow biopsy."

"Oh, no. I am not here for that," I said. "I'm here to get a second opinion."

"Well, that's my opinion," Dr. Ramer said. "You need a bone marrow biopsy. It's the only way you will get a true diagnosis."

I thanked the doctor, paid for my office visit, and left. I continued going to Dr. Uribe for help with the bleeding but never mentioned the high protein in my blood. It was autumn now, and I knew I had to go back home, as I didn't want to spend another winter in Pennsylvania in my condition. I gave my employer notice, made arrangement to see an ENT in Florida, and got my medical reports from the physicians I was seeing. They never knew the extent of my nosebleeds, but then again, no one did. I am a very private person.

As good as it felt to be leaving Pennsylvania, it was also a sad feeling. I was sad because of my health condition and sad because I couldn't let anyone know. I was starting to lose weight, five pounds to be exact, and I didn't know if the weight loss was because of stress or because of the "medical problem."

2

A DIAGNOSIS IS MADE

It was wonderful to be back in Florida, to the home I love and the gardens I'd created for over twenty years. Although I was happy, my illness was always in my thoughts, as I had no idea what the outcome would be. If this was cancer, how sick would I be? Would my world dissolve? Cancer—the word itself is scary! It changes your life; how it changes it is completely up to you, your outlook, and the way you approach life's challenges. But whenever bad thoughts would come, I remembered that God was taking care of me. He was in control.

I made an appointment with the new ENT specialist, Dr. Carri. He thought I should have a surgical cauterization procedure done, after reviewing my medical reports and seeing it had been suggested. He wanted to wait, however, to see how the bleeding progressed. Next, he examined my nostrils. He was shocked to see the scars from so many cauterizations already done and suggested I have a CT scan on my sinus. Again, I didn't mention the high protein in my blood. I guess my thought was if I don't mention anything, it would go away. But it didn't.

A few weeks later, I had a very bad nosebleed, and my ENT, Dr. Carri, was in surgery and couldn't see me. How I missed that little town in Pennsylvania! I called my youngest daughter, who lived nearby at the time, and asked her to take me to the hospital, as I was hesitant to drive myself. My four-year-old granddaughter tagged along. My granddaughter is my best friend. She always wants to be with me. On that trip to the hospital, she would pick at her little nose to make it bleed, and then say, "My nose is bleeding just like Grandma."

At the emergency hospital, the doctor said, "Nosebleeds are a very scary thing."

"I know," I said. "I've been dealing with this for quite a while." He looked inside my nostrils with a scope.

"You're not kidding. Look at all those scars. We'll use a butterfly to stop the bleeding this time." This device, he explained, would have to stay in my nostrils for three to four days before it could be removed. The butterfly looked like a small tampon, a cylindrical bandage with an attached string. The "tampon" goes inside the bleeding nostril, and the string is taped on the cheek—a charming site to behold.

"I suggest your granddaughter leave the room," the doctor said, before he began the procedure. He thought it would be too scary for her. My daughter took my granddaughter by the hand and wished me well as they left the room.

"I want my grandma!" The poor kid went out screaming.

Without warning, the doctor then inserted the "tampon" into my right nostril, with such force that, by reflex, I kicked him. He jerked backward. "I'm sorry," I said, "but you inserted that so hard it feels like it's in the back of my throat."

He started to readjust it, but not before saying, "Don't kick me again."

"I'm sorry," I repeated. "It was not my intention."

Blood was drawn for a CBC—a complete blood panel that gives a picture of your overall health—and I waited for the results. When the results came in about forty-five minutes later, the doctor wanted me to be admitted for more testing. My blood panel had revealed some concerning disorders. I explained to him that my insurance would have to first approve of all these tests he was talking about, and he assured me that since I was admitted to the hospital, it was okay. I chose to believe him. Over the next four days, all sorts of tests were done, including the long-awaited bone marrow biopsy to determine whether or not I had cancer. I was given morphine so I wouldn't feel any pain during the procedure, though the drug had me seeing dragons at every corner, day or night, for almost a year.

Many doctors came in to see me over the next few days. Most of them, I thought, were not needed. On day four, Dr. Carri came in and removed the butterfly from my nostril. At that point, I said, "Enough." I wanted to go home. Leaving the hospital, however, was nowhere near as easy as walking in. A doctor would have to sign papers for my release; I asked Dr. Sanders, the hematology-oncology doctor who was seeing me at the hospital, to do it. I would be following up with her to get the results of the bone marrow biopsy.

I left the hospital that day. The next day, Dr. Sanders's office called to set up an appointment for later that week. I went in, and on that first visit, Dr. Sanders prescribed a medication that I refused. They didn't know what was wrong with me; there had been no diagnosis. I wasn't going to take any unnecessary medications. (Later I found out the medication she was prescribing should not be stopped immediately; I would have had to get off it gradually.) That was strike one against me in her book. More lab tests and an appointment for a CT scan of my chest, abdomen, and pelvis was set up for two weeks later.

In late November 2013, the biopsy results came in, and a diagnosis was made: I had blood cancer. Finding out what was wrong was a relief for me, even though it wasn't the diagnosis I wanted. By then I had already told myself that I did have cancer, so it came as no surprise to hear those words. I was not depressed about it; I finally knew what was wrong and was ready for the battle, with God leading the way. I wasn't feeling pity for myself. I am strong when God is by my side. He would be guiding me.

More tests were done to determine the type of blood cancer it was, which turned out to be Waldenstrom's macroglobulinemia (WM)—a rare white blood cell cancer that is classified as a lymphoplasmacytic lymphoma, a type of B-lymphocyte (B cell) non-Hodgkin's lymphoma. A defining characteristic of this disease is the overproduction of immunoglobulin, the IgM antibodies, which causes the blood to become too thick. Despite advances in research, at this time there is no cure for WM.

Our blood has both a liquid and a solid portion. The liquid portion is the plasma, which contains proteins such as immunoglobulin. In my case, with WM, I had an overproduction of protein in my blood. The liquid portion also contains hormones, albumin, sodium, calcium, and magnesium. Hemoglobin, an iron-containing protein, is found in red blood cells and platelets that help blood to clot. The solid portion of blood contains red blood cells, white blood cells, and platelets. The different types of blood cells perform different duties; the major role of hemoglobin is to carry oxygen from the lungs to the tissues and return carbon dioxide from the tissue to the lungs. It is the oxygen-carrying component of red blood cells. Platelets help blood to clot by bind together when recognizing damaged blood vessels. The white blood cells eliminate bacteria, viruses, and fungi from the body. They also carry out the body immune surveillance and produce, immunoglobulin, which is the IgM I have too much of. White blood cells are found not only in the blood but also in body tissues.

Red blood cells, white blood cells, and platelets develop from blood cells called hematopoietic stem cells. These stem cells can also produce other blood stem cells and are found mainly in the bone marrow, which is a spongy tissue inside our bones. A patient such as myself with WM may not be able to produce some of the different types of blood cells in the bone marrow.

I kept pushing everything on God. "You take care of this, Lord," I prayed. I was very calm knowing God was in control. Prayers were going up to God on my behalf from my church family and from two of my close friends, Tammi and Yasmin, with whom I discussed my illness. Not all my friends and acquaintances knew about the illness. None of my four children could believe what was happening, how sick I was, and at times, they did not want to acknowledge it.

I spent countless hours reading information, educating myself to become familiar with this rare disease and some of the medical terms associated with WM. I wanted to understand more clearly when my physician was explaining my care plan and what to expect from the treatment. The expectation was that the treatments would lower the number of high protein IgM in my blood, the cancer cells. Self-educating allowed me to be my own best advocate.

In December, my nosebleeds were small and far apart, and I went back to work, caring for a wonderful lady I had taken care of for a few years whenever she needed the help. It felt good caring for her. She was a pleasure, and caring for her helped take my mind off my diagnosis. Her family adored me. At one point they noticed that I was a bit thinner and asked me about it. I didn't say, "Oh, I have cancer." It was going to take me some time to get used to saying those words.

Early in January 2014, I received a bill from the hospital. My four-day stay there—and I'd had to insist that I leave on day five—was $29,910.98. My insurance did not pay one penny because of the pre-existing condition clause. I had told the doctors this before they did all those tests, and now the bill was in my lap, and I was responsible for it. A lot of negotiations followed between me and the hospital billing department, which resulted in the bill being reduced to $12,000. Still, that was more than I could afford, with all the other bills coming in from all the doctors that came to my bedside—doctors I did not need. I thought it was highway robbery.

Meanwhile, the recommended treatment plan for my cancer was IV chemotherapy, Cytoxan, for three weeks on and one week off. That would be one chemo session per week for three weeks in a row and the fourth week no chemo. Since this was new to me, I was pretty nervous, to say the least. But as usual, I tried not to show my emotions. I was told that my out-of-pocket cost, including the weekly office visit, would be just over $300. It was a lot of money, but I had to make the financial sacrifice. Once my deductible was met, I would not have a copayment, which was $65 for every doctor visit.

On the way to my first IV chemotherapy treatment, I received a call from a financial counselor at Dr. Sanders' office, advising me that my cost for the treatment would be $200 more because of some pre-meds that had not been included in the total they had quoted me. Instead of $300 per treatment, it was going to be $500 per treatment. That, I could not afford.

At the doctor's office, I sat down with the financial counselor to go over the cost and how I would pay it. She could see that I was a bit frustrated and asked if I would like to speak to Dr. Sanders. "Most definitely," I said, and I sat back as she called for the doctor. I explained to Dr. Sanders that it disturbed me to learn of medications I needed from someone besides herself or her nurse, and going forward I would appreciate that my medications come only from her or her nurse. Strike number two for me in her book. She was not happy. I continued. "Does Cytoxan come orally?" I asked. "I cannot afford it intravenously." She said it did come orally and she wrote me a prescription for it. Now, instead of an IV, I would take one pill a day for ten days, with one week off. This would be about three weeks of chemo for the month. The cost for this would be $78 for the month instead of $1,500. I was relieved. It was a big difference in cost for the same medication, and I didn't have to deal with any IV needles. My chemo treatment went on without much difficulty. My hair didn't fall out; I had very little nausea, too little to take much medication for; and my energy level was good. The biggest problem was that my mouth was very sore. However, a prescribed mouthwash took care of it. My nosebleeds were even shorter and rarer.

My visits with Dr. Sanders started weekly and then went to every other week. In February, lab tests were done, along with exams checking my spleen, lymph nodes, and breasts, and discussion on my overall progress. Preventive medication was prescribed for different side effects from the treatment. Allopurinol was prescribed to prevent gout. After the cancer cells die, the dead cells stay in the bone and can cause gout.

I was working eight to nine hours a day four days a week and feeling good. My IgM was coming down; my Hgb was going up. Great job—things were looking up. As time went on, though, it appeared that my white blood cell count was getting low, which meant I had to be careful of infection. I stayed away from crowds and sick people.

Later that month, at one of my visits with Dr. Sanders, I asked her questions concerning my diagnosis. She was very annoyed. "If I answer all your questions, I won't have time to see other patients," she said. "You should trust me. I have fourteen years of experience in this field. Well, I was certainly not expecting that response from her, and I told her so.

"I thought your job was to answer all your patients' questions," I said.

"You question every management plan and have refused to take some medications. Noncompliance is an issue that might interfere with your medical care."

"Patients do have the right to refuse medications," I reminded her.

We parted on good terms, with smiles and a handshake. Driving home, I reasoned with myself. Maybe I should find another doctor. Maybe I did ask too many questions. But how else would I learn about my disease? The doctor is the one that I should be asking, not Google. Then again, Google didn't get upset no matter how many questions I ask. Patients are not inclined to question their doctors because some have an invisible barrier around them that can be intimidating. I went back to Dr. Sanders for a few more visits, and when I had a question, I asked it.

On Sunday, March 21, 2014, I noticed blood in my urine. I felt somewhat frantic because it was a Sunday and Dr. Sanders's office was closed, but there is a twenty-four-hour on-call physician for emergencies, so I left a message and asked for someone to return my call. In about fifteen minutes I received a call back from the on-call physician, Dr. Jay. I explained my problem and was told to stop taking the chemo medication; the bleeding was a severe side effect from it. He advised me to call the office on Monday for an appointment with Dr. Sanders and get a urine culture and a lab test. Early Monday morning, at 8:30 a.m. to be exact, I made the call. Dr. Sanders was not in, so I left word for her to please call me so I could make an appointment to see her and get urine and lab tests. Late that afternoon, the office called with the appointment for the test the following day. I never heard from Dr. Sanders or her nurse.

The following day I was sitting in the lab area, just about to have blood drawn, when my nose began bleeding. Blood gushed down my face, was even streaming down my throat. It was a horrible mess. I was petrified, too frightened to move. The nurse that was about to draw my blood was startled and gave me gauze pads to keep the blood from getting all over me and the floor; it didn't help. The blood just kept coming. Needless to say, no labs were done that day. My ENT, Dr. Carri, was in the same building, so I went there for help, only to learn that he didn't take my insurance anymore. He was one of many doctors who opted out of ACA and refused to see patients with this plan. I asked if I could self-pay. "We'll get back to you. He is in surgery," the receptionist replied, while I stood in front of her with an uncontrollable bloody nose.

I was frustrated. Here, I needed immediate medical attention but could not receive it because of the bureaucracy going on between the doctors and the ACA. Doctors, I believe, should always remember the medical oath of good judgment and use it more often. That day, I called several other ENTs for help, telling them that I would self-pay, but their fee ranged between $900 and $1,200, which I could not afford.

Back to the hospital I went, seeking that awful butterfly to stop the bleeding. I was there for three hours, and my copay was $150. With my ACA coverage, the first visit to the emergency room was $150. The second visit would be about $650, a price meant to discourage patients with nonemergencies from going to the ER. Patients are instead encouraged to go to urgent care. Sadly, I never heard from my oncologist, Dr. Sanders. After the way she treated me, I could not trust her anymore. I realized I should have walked away from her some time ago.

Three weeks after this event with the nosebleed and the sudden stopping of the chemo, I got a call from Dr. Sanders's office, telling me to come in for a visit because she would be leaving soon for vacation. I explained that I would not see Dr. Sanders anymore because I didn't think she had my best interest in mind, and I asked for all my medical records. I was scared and didn't know what I would do now or how I would find a physician that would give me the care I so desperately needed. By now I had been off chemo for a month. How was I supposed to go about finding a new doctor? I spoke with someone I knew with a blood disorder, and she referred me to her physician. At my appointment with the new physician, I became aware that he could not help me, and he also knew it. He knew nothing about WM. He told me the group of doctors I came from were the best. My hopes were dashed.

3

MY NEW ONCOLOGIST

A few days later a friend called, telling me that the Leukemia Lymphoma Society had a program that helps with copay assistance for those who qualify. *Well, that is not what I need right now*, I thought. I needed an oncologist-hematologist. But I took the information and made the call. When the receptionist answered, instead of asking about copay assistance, I said, "Do you know of an oncology physician who treats Waldenstrom's patients?"

"I don't," she replied, "but there is someone volunteering in this office that is living with WM. Leave your information, and she will give you a call." I was interested and eager.

A day later the woman called. I explained my situation to her and how I felt I was not being treated adequately by my former physician. This surprised her. She went to the same group of doctors and was being treated by a different one, Dr. Jacobson. She liked this doctor very much. She told me to let him know that she referred me. I appreciated the referral, but at the same time, I did not want to go back to the same group of doctors. I didn't want to ever go back to that building. My experience there was so horrible; it took several weeks for me to even drive down the street the building is on. I was amazed by how cancer patients can be treated, with very little empathy or respect. As a healthcare provider, myself, I treat all my patients with respect and empathy.

I honor their dignity. If I weren't a strong person, the way I had been treated so far would have left me demoralized. As a cancer patient, I felt I was just a money machine for some physicians. Sad as it is to say, from my perspective, not much compassion is given. But I needed a doctor, and a good one, and this woman had a lot of faith in Dr. Jacobson. I wanted to give him a chance. I did a little research and found out there were three locations for his medical practice, which gave me hope. The location I'd gone to was only ten minutes away, but I would gladly drive the extra twenty minutes to the second location.

On Monday, April 28, 2014, I called Dr. Jacobson's office to make an appointment. To my surprise, I hit a brick wall.

"You cannot see Dr. Jacobson," the receptionist told me, "since you've been seen by another physician in the practice." She had to be kidding! I had no idea this was the protocol with the medical profession—another road block, one more hurdle for me to get over. All my life I had struggled; I had been knocked down, and I had always gotten back up. Why should this be any different?

"Dr. Jacobson advertised he was accepting new patients, and I am a new patient to him," I said.

"You are not a new patient to this group. I'm sorry," the receptionist said.

A cancer diagnosis was not part of my life plan, and fighting to see a physician was not on my to-do list.

"I am a very sick person," I told her, "and I am being penalized for leaving a physician that did not have my best interest at heart. This is my life we are discussing."

"Okay," the woman said. "I will put in the request, but the two physicians—Dr. Sanders and Dr. Jacobson—will have to agree. You'll get a call after the doctors' discussion." Two weeks later I had an appointment to see Dr. Jacobson. It is unbelievable what people like me should go through just trying to get adequate medical care. All patients deserve quality and affordable care.

My friendships during this time were also giving me some

unexpected surprises. I was realizing that many of the people I had considered my friends were casually disappearing after learning of my cancer diagnosis. It was as if I was contagious. I received very few phone calls, and some of those who called and asked to have lunch with me never showed up. Now I knew without question who my real friends were. One of them was a dear brother in Christ who was also going through a cancer journey. Even with what he was going through, he thought of others. One day I received a card from him in the mail. Later that same day, an email came in from our church, saying that my friend had passed away that day. "Oh, my goodness," I thought, "I just received his card today. He was saying good-bye to me."

Late Wednesday afternoon, May 14, 2014, I waited in Dr. Jacobson's office, eager to meet him and get started. I had been without treatment for nearly ten weeks, and I was not feeling so well. I had extremely bad headaches, and my neck was stiff. I desperately needed a physician, and a good one.

Dr. Jacobson gave a quick knock on the exam room door, walked in, shook my hand, and introduced himself. He was polite, soft-spoken, and had a nice smile. "So, what was the problem with Dr. Sanders?" he asked. I wasn't expecting that question and was hesitant to tell him my true experiences with Dr. Sanders.

"I was not happy with the care I was receiving," I simply said, hoping that would be enough. It seemed to be.

Dr. Jacobson's exam was thorough. My lymph nodes were not swollen, but the doctor was concerned about the stiffness in my neck. I told him about my headaches and other things that concerned me. My next appointment would be in one week, he said, and he would have a treatment plan for us to go over at that time. He called prescriptions for my headache and the stiffness in my neck into my pharmacy. I left the cancer center feeling energized. It was a good feeling to be getting back in the saddle and treating my disease.

4

MY TREATMENT PLAN

At that time, there was no medication approved by the FDA that was specifically for WM. Therefore, all the medications I would receive were trials to see what would help. I trusted Dr. Jacobson and believed he had my best interests in mind and would be doing everything he could possibly do. He believed strongly in helping his patients make good decisions, by explaining the options that were available. I could ask him any question regarding my care, and his answers were always helpful.

I was glad the woman I was caring for was away all summer, because there was no way I could have worked once I started Dr. Jacobson's cancer treatment plan. For about three months, there would be one weekly intravenous chemotherapy drug, along with Rituxan, followed by a lab test and an examination in Dr. Jacobson's office. After a few months, we would have more information and know more about how to proceed.

On June 4, 2014, I went into the chemotherapy area—the infusion room—feeling anxious. I didn't know what to expect. I had heard and read that the chemo drug I was to receive could produce severe side effects during the application of it, and I would be carefully monitored by the nurse for the entire five-hour procedure. My daughter and granddaughter drove me to the cancer center that day and would be there to pick me up when the treatment was finished, five hours later. When the nurse saw me, with a kind expression in her eyes, she said, "You look scared."

"I am," I told her. "This is my first chemotherapy infusion." She assured me she would be right by my side.

"Everything will be fine," she said. She explained the procedures and said that at the first sign of a side effect, she would either stop the process or slow it down. I nodded, settling into my reclining chair. Gently and professionally, she inserted the IV needle into my arm; there was little discomfort. She gave me the pre-meds, which were slightly sedative, followed by the chemo medication. By now I was feeling drowsy from the pre-meds, and I fell asleep for most of the procedure. Five and a half hours later, my first chemo treatment was done. My daughter and granddaughter met me as planned, but I could see it was going to be possible for me to leave on my own after future treatments. I wasn't too weak from the chemo to drive. After that first treatment, for the next four days I had no energy. I felt weak and tired. My hair was thinner, and I had some slight nausea. I took medication for side effects, such as nausea, which helped. And then, just when my body was starting to recover, it was time for my second treatment.

June continued with more chemo treatments, but the high protein count in my blood (IgM) didn't come down. In July, there were no chemo treatments, just weekly visits to Dr. Jacobson and more lab tests. I came down with bronchitis and was given an intravenous drug to support my immune system. From August through October 2014, two new chemotherapy drugs, Treanda and Valcade, were tried, and I was given numerous blood tests, which were essential for my physician to see if these new drugs were working. In November and December, my treatment regimens were the same: I was at the cancer center eight to nine days out of the month for several hours each time, I saw my doctor regularly, and I had one treatment after the other. Lab tests, injections for my white blood cells, infusions to support my immune system, and of course, the chemotherapy sessions continued. I felt like a pin cushion, though I was not complaining, as the cancer center became my second home, where everyone knew my name.

The year 2015 began, and my treatment plan stayed the same, but there was little difference in my cancer. The IgM was still very high. Dr. Jacobson suggested another bone marrow biopsy. He had noticed something in the first report that he thought needed a second look. I wasn't too happy about it because the biopsy had to be done at the cancer center instead of at the hospital, where I could receive a stronger drug to block the pain of the procedure. Nevertheless, as I said before, I trusted Dr. Jacobson immensely, and I agreed to go forward.

On February 2 one of Dr. Jacobson's nurses explained the procedure. Dr. Jacobson came in and proceeded with the bone marrow biopsy. He sliced my flesh to insert the needle that would enter my bone to retrieve some marrow for the biopsy. In the middle of the procedure, he asked me how I was doing. I said, "Okay," but I was thinking, "How could I be okay with this big needle grinding into my bone?" Before long, it was over, and the doctor showed me what he had taken out for the test. It didn't look like much for all I had to endure, but it was over, and I was ready to get out of there and go home. First, though, I had to get chemo, so I went to the infusion room for my treatment. After a gruesome and tiring day, I finally got home about five hours later. Two weeks later, at my appointment with Dr. Jacobson, I was happy to learn he was very pleased with the results of the bone marrow biopsy. It was not what he had suspected, so all was well.

In March 2015, the FDA approved Imbrutinib, the first medication for WM. As expected, it was very expensive, but my insurance paid for it. Dr. Jacobson was optimistic, as so far nothing was working. I was quite relieved that the medication was in pill form and not to be taken intravenously. I started taking Imbrutinib orally on Tuesday, March 24, and two days later, it appeared to me that there was blood in my stool. I spoke to Dr.

Jacobson's nurse about what I was seeing, and after discussing it with Dr. Jacobson, she told me to go directly to the hospital. He would tell them to expect me and instruct them about my care.

When I arrived at the hospital, a test was done, but they found no blood in the stool. I was given platelets because my platelet count was very low, and when there is a low platelet count, blood has a difficult time clotting to stop bleeding. I was not feeling sick and was ready to leave at that point, but the doctors recommended I stay overnight for observation. I politely declined. A couple more doctors came to see me, curious to know why I did not want to stay. I restated that I was not feeling sick. They told me they were not the police and could not keep me, but suggested I wait until they spoke to Dr. Jacobson. Four hours later, discharge papers were drawn up, and I was free to go. The following morning, I called Dr. Jacobson to tell him I hadn't stayed at the hospital, which I know he knew, but I was being polite. I reminded him our next appointment was in five days, but he wanted to see me right away. "Come in immediately," he said. "Well, not immediately, but sometime today." Later that day, Dr. Jacobson examined me and said that even though the hospital test did not show it, there might have been bleeding and to stop taking the Imbrutinib. In two weeks, I was back to taking the first chemo drug he prescribed nearly a year before, Rituxan.

I was feeling good, even though my IgM was high and most of my lab tests were not good. The last big nosebleed I'd had was on March 21, 2014. My energy level was good most of the time, and I had no bad reactions from all the chemo I was taking. Life was good! I still wasn't able to return to work because I wasn't strong enough, and I was afraid of getting sick because of my low white blood cell count. I continued eating healthy meals, lots of fruits and vegetables and fish and soups. I'm not sure if it made any difference, but I read somewhere that blueberries were good for helping with low platelets, so I ate more blueberries than usual. I read that garlic and onions have antioxidants that help protect against cancer; I started eating lots of garlic and onions with my scrambled eggs.

I am a very creative person, however, with this disease, it was hard to do many of the things I did for many years and loved, like painting, decoupage, and garden design. I did lots of seashell designs on wood, mirrors, picture frames, and chandeliers. Many of my creative designs were sold in high-end stores. Now I could not tolerate the smells of perfumes, paints, or any other strong odors. Smells like these, for some reason, would trigger a nosebleed. Besides not being strong enough to do the creative crafts I did when I was a creative entrepreneur, I couldn't even practice my healthcare profession, which I also loved. I felt like I was peeking at the world I knew from inside a bubble. I desperately needed to transform myself.

One gloomy, rainy day, because of the weather conditions, I left home earlier than usual for an appointment with Dr. Jacobson. I arrived about thirty minutes early, so I went to the cafeteria for a cup of my favorite soup, clam chowder. The cafeteria was on the north side ground level of this five-story hospital building. The upper stories are medical offices, a chapel, and the cancer center. The smells walking into the cafeteria were delicious; I hurried over to get my soup. I couldn't wait to have a taste. I sat down at a table for four in front of a window to enjoy my soup; there was no wind blowing, no rustling leaves, just rain.

I was looking at the traffic coming in and going out, when a nicely dressed man came up and said, "May I join you?" Before I could answer, he pulled a chair and took a seat, his back to the window, blocking my view. He extended his hand and said, "I'm Ron." He introduced himself with a distinctive burst of energy and a big smile, like he was pleased to see me. Ron looked to be about 175 lbs, 6' 2" maybe, and about in his late fifties, with curly brown hair and a light brown complexion. He was wearing a long-sleeve peach shirt with gray pants. He said he was frequently in the building and had seen me on several occasions. "I wave, but you never seem to notice."

"My mind is always somewhere else," I told him. "Don't take it personally." We talked briefly about the pouring rain, and then I saw it was time for me to leave. "It was nice talking with you," I said, standing, "but I have an appointment."

"What did you say your name is?" he asked.

"I didn't say," I told him, smiling. His body language now showed disappointment. Off to my appointment I went, thinking, "*Wow!* Someone actually, noticed me." I wondered if he would still want to have a chat if he knew of my dilemma.

Four weeks later, on May 5, 2015, a CT scan of my chest, abdomen, and pelvis was performed. Leaving my doctor's office, I saw the nicely dressed man, Ron, walking down the hallway. He waved. "How was your soup today?"

"I didn't have any," I replied.

"And your name is?" he asked.

"Elsie," I said.

"I used to have an Aunt Elsie, but she died a hundred years ago," he said, laughing.

"Don't remind me it's an old name," I said, smiling.

"I'm on a mission right now, so you have a good afternoon 'Aunt Elsie,'" and with that, he rushed off. As I was driving home, I was thinking about Ron. He seemed like a nice person, with lots of energy, and he had a nice sense of humor. I liked that. I liked people who could make me laugh without trying. I wanted to get to know him. Who was he, and why was he so often at the cancer center? I decided to wait for him to tell me; showing my curiosity would only give him a chance to ask me things I may not want to discuss.

No chemotherapy treatment was given for May and June. I was getting lab tests done and weekly neuprogen injections for my white blood cells. On July 13 I started another chemotherapy, an orally administered drug called Revlimid, at 5 mg. At first my insurance company denied payment for this drug, as it was not approved for my diagnosis. Somehow, though, Dr. Jacobson did it, and the drug company gave me the medication monthly. The treatment plan was three pills per week, two weeks on and one week off.

By now about six weeks had passed since I had seen Ron, and I began to think I probably wouldn't see him again, but three weeks later, there he was coming out of an office as I was heading to the elevator. He did not see me, as he was busy looking down at some papers he was carrying. "Hello, stranger," I said. "Haven't seen you in a while." He looked up from the papers.

"Oh, hi, Elsie." He smiled. "You look as beautiful as this gorgeous day." I couldn't help but smile as his energy erupted.

"Do you have time for coffee? Iced tea?" I said, and we walked together to the cafeteria.

When we took our drinks to sit at a table, I saw him notice the blisters that had formed on my arms from the medication I was taking. He gently touched my arm. "You have sensitive skin," he said. He told me he had been away for a couple of months, but he didn't say why.

"Well, I'm glad you're back," I said. "It's nice to see a friendly face in this building now and then."

"You're right. There are a lot of serious faces around here, and then there's mine," he said, grinning.

"Don't flatter yourself." I laughed. Just then, Ron's cell phone rang.

"Let's do this again," he said, and in a flash, he was off, his coffee cup still half-full. I wished he had asked for my phone number; I would have liked to see him again, and outside of the medical building. The cancer journey can be very lonely, and human contact is important. I appreciated his calm demeanor. He was so easy to talk to. I felt as if we had known each other a long time.

Revlimid was hard on my system, but it was the first medication to show signs of helping reduce the cancer in my blood. The IgM was finally going down. I had a terrible rash—itchy blisters all over my body—which puzzled Dr. Jacobson. He suggested I see a dermatologist, which I did. I saw Dr. Brien, who performed a biopsy that confirmed the medication was the cause of the rash. Cream, ointment, and a lotion were prescribed to be used as needed for the rash. By mid-August, because of this side effect, the dose was reduced to two pills per week, with no off week. This dosage, however, did not perform as well, so Dr. Jacobson put me back on three pills per week. I think I had almost all the side effects associated with this drug, but I tolerated them because this drug was doing very well in destroying the high protein count; my IgM was going down, and my platelet count was up. I was very excited. Finally, something was working.

There were a couple of scares along the way, however. On September 23, I went to see my ophthalmologist, Dr. Zell, because that morning I had lost vision in my right eye for about twenty minutes. He found nothing but said it must have been a small blood clot moving around my eye that morning. He spoke with Dr. Jacobson regarding the eye test, and Dr. Jacobson wanted further testing done. He scheduled for me to have a Vascular Studies Carotid Doppler, on both sides. Using ultrasound, this test would check the blood flow in my neck to be sure there was not a blockage there, causing me to lose vision. This test was done on September 28. The tests did not show any blockage, and I continued taking the chemo medication, Revlimid, with all its side effects.

A few months later Ron asked if I would like to have lunch at a little restaurant not far from the cancer center. I told him sure; I'd meet him there. As he was giving me directions, I realized he was describing Burger King, a block away. "Burger King?!" I said. "No, thank you."

"I'm kidding!" He laughed. He gave me the right directions this time, to a small restaurant just up the street.

A little bit later, we were seated at the restaurant, where I ordered a bowl of lobster bisque." No burger for you?" Ron said, smiling.

"Funny guy," I thought.

He told me he worked for a pharmaceutical company, which kept him busy. "My life is quite complicated," he said, "but it's always a treat running into you."

"That's nice," I said. "You're good company." I learned that day that Ron was unmarried and was caring for his deceased sister's child, who has a chronic medical condition. I was surprised and saddened to learn of his circumstances, though I thought that taking on such responsibility showed his courage, strength, and humility. In life, you never know what's around the corner. Important people can show up in unexpected places and at unexpected times. Sometimes we can meet amazing, sweet people like Ron. I looked forward to our meetings. They give me hope and reinforcement. For me, they were like little vacation islands in my life.

5

MEDICATION-INDUCED ACUTE HEPATITIS B: LIVER FAILURE

In mid-October 2015, I started back to my caregiver work, and all was going well. Four months later, on February 8, Dr. Jacobson said that my IgM looked very good. He said I was healthy, confirming how I felt. Blood was drawn for a lab test, and I was given a chemo treatment with Rituxan, the medication I took the first time I had intravenous chemotherapy. I left the cancer center that day, feeling very upbeat.

But surprises were right around the corner. The very next day, Dr. Jacobson called, telling me to go immediately to the emergency room at the hospital. My blood test the day before showed that my bilirubin was extremely high. Bilirubin is a reddish-yellow substance that is produced during the normal breakdown of old red blood cells. High bilirubin means there may be a problem involving the red blood cells, liver, or gallbladder. Dr. Jacobson suspected a problem with my gallbladder. A surgeon and a doctor were expecting me, he said.

"Can this wait until tomorrow morning?" I asked. "I'm on my way to work."

"No, go immediately." I called my employer to tell her of my emergency, and then off I went to the hospital.

"I'm having surgery," I said to myself. I had never had one of those. I wondered how long I would have to be in the hospital. Cancer is such an unsteady hand. Yesterday Dr. Jacobson had said I was healthy, and today, apparently, I was not. It didn't matter how healthy I was feeling; something could be changing. I just couldn't be too comfortable; a shadow was always lurking.

While driving to the hospital I looked back on the last three or four days and realized I was feeling a little nauseous, but I hadn't thought much of it. My urine was a bit darker than usual, but I had thought it was from not drinking enough water. I had been so busy at work that I wasn't paying much attention to my well-being. Nevertheless, I wasn't feeling sick.

When I arrived at the hospital, sure enough, the doctors were there, ready to pounce on me. A nurse checked me in, and the surgeon came over to see me. "I looked at the reports Dr. Jacobson sent," the surgeon said, "and I don't think you are having an operation today. I saw a tiny spot on your gallbladder, but it doesn't mean an operation is necessary."

"Good news," I said. I was put in a room, and blood was drawn for some tests. An ultrasound was done to check on my gallbladder. In a few hours, I was sent home.

The following day, Dr. Jacobson recommended I have another test done. I went in to have another ultrasound and a CT scan of my abdomen. After reviewing the information, Dr. Jacobson told me I had acute hepatitis B and liver failure induced by medication. Liver failure is one of the severe side effects of Revlimid, the one chemotherapy drug that was working well in bringing down my cancer. I saw that Dr. Jacobson was very concerned about what was happening, as my liver lab reports were through the roof. A normal bilirubin range is 0.2 to 1.2; mine was 35 and rising. I was told there were no medications for this problem; the liver would heal itself.

I was devastated. Just as I was feeling better, this happened. I felt defeated, but I wasn't going to crumble. I dug deep down and found the strength I never knew I had. I believed and trusted in my oncologist, and I could see he was quite worried about me. Maybe he said this to calm me and give me hope, but he told me that in his forty years of practice, he had seen only two other cases of this happening and both had turned out well.

I quit my job to start fighting this disease. We all have something in our lives that we wish we could change. I remember telling myself not to give up; God was bigger than this, and would not let me down.

Dr. Jacobson collaborated with colleagues who were liver specialists, and these doctors worked together to help control my devastating problem. I love Valentine's Day and all the chocolate that comes with it. But on Valentine's Day 2016, instead of chocolate, I was given medication: Lamvudine 300 mg, one pill daily to keep my liver failure in the acute stage and not let it go into a chronic condition. Two weeks later, the Lamvudine was switched to Viread 300 mg, once daily, which was then switched to Entecavir 0.5 mg, once daily.

I was exhausted. With liver failure, I felt much worse than I had with the effects of any chemotherapy treatment. I cannot find words to describe just how extremely weak and exhausted I was feeling. I thought it was inhumane to be as sick as I was, with no medication to alleviate my discomfort. When I told Dr. Jacobson this, he ordered five weeks of bed rest. My abdomen was starting to extend from accumulated fluid I was retaining, the whites of my eyes were yellow from jaundice, my stool was a light gray, and the color of my urine was very dark orange. I was getting all sorts of lab tests two times a week, and my arms were badly bruised from the blood draws. My feet and toes were swollen, and it was difficult to walk. I was a total mess. But it's always been hard for me to show my true emotions. I kept going with a smile.

On an elevator at the hospital one day, I noticed a young man staring at me. That was not unusual, because of my physical appearance and condition. Finally, he said, "Do you have sickle cell disease?"

"No," I told him. "Your eyes are yellow. Check with your doctor.

"Don't add another problem," I said to myself. I was glad when the elevator doors opened, and I could get out.

I was born in the 1950s and was three years old when my mother died giving birth to my youngest sibling, who died with her. I believe that day was the beginning of many difficulties, and the start of my willpower to overcome them all. I was the second to last child, with four older siblings. My father practically raised us all on his own. He was a very caring dad, but he didn't have the touch a mother has. The experience of that deep mother's love is something I always yearned for. I have often wondered about my mom, how it must have been so hard for her, knowing she was dying and leaving her children behind, her babies.

I have a long-ago memory of the event. I was a little girl, and there was a procession with so many people all around. I was so happy to see them all. I thought I was in some sort of celebration. I wondered where my mother was. Why wasn't she here? I didn't understand it was her funeral I was attending.

Until I was about five years old, I cried a lot. I don't know why I did; I just know I would sit and cry for no apparent reason. It must have been because I missed my mother. I don't recall any of us asking about her, and I have no memories of my father talking about her. The only person who always spoke about my mother was my mother's brother, my uncle. He would say to us kids, "How I wish your father had died instead of your mother." My uncle despised my dad. He blamed my father for my mother's death. According to him, before my mother got pregnant that last time, the doctor had told my parents it would be life threatening for my mother to have another child because she had a chronic problem with anemia. As a young child, I did not understand any of this. I felt bad for my dad and for the grief my uncle was experiencing. My siblings and I stayed away from our uncle as much as possible, as we didn't like how he would constantly depreciate our father. I wanted him to stop.

After I turned five, I saw crying as a sign of weakness, and I believed I must be strong always. I knew my family was strong and capable; we could carry ourselves. Even when my heart was breaking, I never let anyone know what was bothering me. When obstacles came my way, I did everything in my power to overcome them, and I did it always with a smile. Whenever I was knocked down and my knees were scraped, I got up and brushed it off like nothing had happened. I didn't have many friends as a young child; I didn't want to let anyone get too close to me and know much about me. I was extremely introverted. I also had a speech impediment. (I had that until I was about nine years old.) It was difficult for me to pronounce certain words properly. "Medicine" was one of the words that I finally mastered in my late teens.

People would try to take advantage of me, thinking I couldn't defend myself. They would notice that I observed more than I verbalized. But I always stood up for myself. People seemed amazed to learn that I did have a voice and could use it.

Because friends wanted to know more than I was willing to share with them, I believed it was best to have as few friends as possible. My siblings were different. They had many friends and thought I was a bit strange.

As a child, my friends were older people. I loved older people— grandparents, and people of that age. They were always pleasant and had funny stories to tell. There was one sweet old gentleman, a neighbor of ours named Mr. Toby. Mr. Toby was the cutest little old man I knew. I loved Mr. Toby. He had chubby cheeks, wore an old-fashioned hat, and walked with a stick. He was a bundle of joy, always smiling and happy to see us. He would often bring us cookies or banana bread he had made. He would sit and chat with us kids, telling the same stories on every visit. I didn't mind; I loved it. My sisters and brother would take their goodies and dash off, holding their noses. I, on the other hand, always sat and talked with him, wondering how I could get him to smell better. I loved him so much that I named my first pet Mr. Toby.

Twenty years after I lost my mother, my father died. My siblings and I were very sad, but we didn't show our tears. By now we were professionals at suppressing our feelings. For most of our lives we had suffered tremendously, from one tragedy after the next. When I was six years old, my eldest sister, Miriam, died trying to save my cousin, my uncle's son, from drowning; they both drowned. We were devastated. Miriam was like a mother to us, and it felt like losing our mother twice. Four years later, when I was ten years old, my second oldest sister died from typhoid fever. We had so much hurt so young; we became skillful with cutting ourselves off from feeling more pain.

By the time I was forty-five years old, I had lost all my siblings to different diseases. There were heart problems; there was diabetes. I would have loved to have one of them with me now, but I reassured myself that God was in control, He would get me through this.

My strong spiritual background comes from my father, who was raised Catholic. He prayed with us every day and reminded us that God loves us and will protect us. My father memorized many chapters of the bible (I thought he was such a smart man to do this), and he always studied it with us. We regularly attended Mass. I believed strongly that there was a God and that He would give us what we needed, but as I grew, I wasn't getting satisfaction from the Mass. I began to have questions about the rosary beads and making confession to a man instead of going directly to God, I spoke with my dad about my feelings and told him I wanted to visit a church not too far from our neighborhood to see how they worship. He agreed to it, and I went. Right away I felt so much closer to God, as if he were my best friend. I could speak to him directly at any time. I worshipped at that church on a regular basis, gaining a sense of security and community. Those feelings helped me then as they helped me now, sustaining me through the challenges I faced.

Now that I had liver failure on top of the cancer, I was gaining about eight pounds a week—all of it from fluid retention. I asked Dr. Jacobson for something to help eliminate some of the fluid, and he suggested what he called an endovascular procedure, where fluid is drawn out by a large needle at the end of a tube that is inserted into the abdomen. I made the appointment with a physician they called "an interventional oncology physician."

Before I saw the doctor for the procedure, I saw Ron one day at the cancer center. My body was showing the effects of my liver failure. I was not feeling well. Ron was concerned. "Be sure to call if you need any help," he said, and he gave me his phone number. I did call on him a few times, and he was helpful in finding ways to alleviate some of my health difficulties.

I underwent the painful procedure for the fluid draw three times with this doctor. Unfortunately, however, the fluid returned each time in under three hours. The doctor suggested we try a procedure he called "insert abdomen-venus drain," where a shunt is inserted into the abdomen and stays there, draining fluid off to various organs. It would be doing some of the job of the liver until that organ was functioning well again. This physician had done this procedure many times, he said, with great success. There was only a 1 percent rejection rate.

I discussed the procedure with Dr. Jacobson and decided to go ahead with it. It was an outpatient procedure and would be completed in two hours. I would be released from the hospital five hours after having it. "Bring someone to drive you home," the doctor nurse advised, so I asked a friend, who agreed to help me out. My appointment was for 12:30 p.m. on April 12, and I planned to arrive two hours early, as they suggested.

6

VERY DRAMATIC

On April 12, I arrived at the hospital on time, checked in, and all was going well. The anesthesiologist came in and introduced herself. She explained the type of anesthesia I would be getting and described what would happen during the procedure. She said there might be a tube placed in my mouth to assist with my breathing during the procedure, but the doctor would make that determination as the procedure progressed. She asked if I had any questions, and I did not. It sounded very straightforward. I wasn't afraid, and I was ready to get started.

The anesthesiologist left the room and returned a short time later, saying the doctor wanted the tube to be put in at the beginning of the procedure. He would be in shortly. She then administered the anesthesia, which took immediate effect. I was totally out. I did not know when the doctor came, and I felt nothing of what was done.

When I woke after the procedure, I had quite a surprise. It was the next day, April 13! "Why am I still in the hospital?" I wondered. "What happened?" I was supposed to be able to go home after five hours the same day. I was drowsy and incoherent. The friend who planned to take me home came in to see me. "Do you know why I'm still here?" I asked her. She did not. She said the doctor kept pushing the time back for me to leave and had finally said I would stay over.

Besides my friend, there was no one else in my room. A nurse's aide came in. I later learned from my friend that I had been sliding off my pillow and wanted help getting back up on it so I had called for a nurse. I knew from my experience as a caregiver that one person cannot get this done efficiently with a person in my condition; two persons were needed. Yet, here was my CNA, and he was alone. He removed a portion of the blanket covering me, and I heard my friend say, with alarm, "Oh my, she is bleeding!" At that, the CNA ran out the room. A few nurses ran in. My friend left the room. I must have passed out, because when I opened my eyes I was back in the area of the hospital where the procedure had been done the day before. The nurses were frantic. I was bleeding profusely from the incisions the doctor had made to insert the shunt. My body was rejecting it, and I was in tremendous pain. One of them asked if I could slide over onto a bed that was pushed next to whatever I was lying on. I couldn't understand why they didn't just push me in on the bed that I was on in the room, but I said nothing and tried to do as she asked. As I attempted to raise myself to slide over on the bed, I heard myself scream in pain, though it sounded like it was coming from somewhere else. I had never in my life scream that loud before. "What's the matter?" I heard a nurse yell. "What's wrong?"

"I cannot breathe! I cannot breathe!" It was hard to get the words out.

"Calm down," she said. "Take a deep breath. This good-looking young man will put an oxygen mask on you."

The anesthesiologist was there and without a word gave me anesthesia. I was fading, but still conscious enough to hear the nurse calling for the physician, but he was apparently not answering. She kept repeating it: "He is not answering!"

"Call his cell phone," I suggested. I could not believe that this doctor could not be reached at this critical time. I was sure another doctor would help as I lay waiting for what felt like an eternity.

She told me again, "He is not answering."

"Please call my oncologist, Dr. Jacobson," I said. That is the last thing I remember before the anesthesia took full effect and I was out.

When I woke up, I was in the intensive care unit. My friend came in and asked how I was feeling. "I'm not sure," I told her. "I know I've had better days." We chuckled about that. My daughter came in next, which surprised me because she lived out of state. I hadn't mentioned to her that I was having this procedure done, as I thought it was no big deal, just an outpatient procedure. She said she had come unannounced to see me, as a surprise. As soon as she'd gotten in, she'd learned that I was in the hospital. "Well, it is so good to see you," I said. "You came just in time."

While I was explaining what had happened, a friend from my church walked into the room. "Elsie!" she said. "What is going on?"

I had no idea how in the world this friend knew I was in the hospital. I hadn't even known I was going to be here. I explained to her briefly what had happened, and soon after that, she left. Before I knew it, another visitor came by. I was still wondering how all these people knew what was going on, but I was happy to see them all. Later that day the doctor came by.

"Elsie," he said, standing close to my bed and looking into my eye, "remember I told you I have done this procedure many times with great success and that there was a 1 percent rejection rate? Well, you are it." With that, he smiled, patted the bed, and left.

Bandages covered the right side of my body, from my shoulder to my hip. My abdomen was still extended from the accumulation of fluid. I remained in ICU a few more days, with fluid being drawn out twice more and with Dr. Jacobson at my side twice daily, managing my care. I received lots of blood, platelets, and other medication to clot my blood. On the third day, I was out of intensive care and in a regular room.

Very early the morning of April 18, Dr. Jacobson came in to see me. "I want to go home," I told him. I'd had enough of the hospital—more than enough. He was astonished.

"You want to go home? Okay, I'll get the papers ready so you can leave." Before I went home that day, I asked to see the physician that did the procedure so my bandages could be changed and he could see the progress of the wound healing. It was obvious I was in pain, and he apologized.

"Come back and see me in ten days, and I'll remove the stitches," he said. I said I would, and I left for home. It wasn't easy going home. I was not as strong as I had thought I was. A couple of steps and I was exhausted. I could barely raise my right arm, and it was very difficult getting into the car. But I was happy to be out of the hospital.

At home, things were worse instead of better. My bed turned out to be too high to get into, so I went to my couch. Trying to get up from there was a nightmare. I was too weak to raise myself and get my feet on the floor. I am right-handed, and my right arm was not functioning due to the operation, and using my left arm was exhausting. I needed assistance. My daughter, who was still in town, stayed on to help me. It was hard asking for assistance every five minutes or so, very frustrating. I purchased a lift recliner, the kind that assists with getting up to a standing position, but it did not work for me because the feet section was low. A pillow was placed under my legs to elevate and help with the fluid retention, however I had no strength to get the pillow under my legs or take it out without help. The recliner was returned in a couple of days, and I went back to lying on the couch. For about two weeks, I couldn't do much for myself. Even holding a cup in my right hand was impossible; my hand would shake terribly, and I would spill whatever was in it. Friends visited. One of them was Tina, my very special Romanian friend. Tina recommended a home remedy from her country. She gathered some Chinese cabbage leaf and wrapped my abdomen with it, saying the cabbage should take the fluid out. I slept wrapped with the cabbage leaf for a few nights, and it did not work. Today, we are still laughing about it.

It became clear to me I was not a good patient. Everyone was getting fed up with me, and my calls for help sometimes went unanswered. I was very sick, feeling awful, and was projecting my feelings of pain and discomfort onto others, people who were there to help me. Once I realized this and identified the emotions that I was projecting, I apologized to my daughter and I told her she could leave whenever she wanted. I had been home for three weeks, and though my right arm was still not functioning, I felt that I could do enough for myself. I imagine my daughter felt like doing cartwheels. She left the next day. Looking back over all that had transpired with my health so far, I knew that God was caring for me through it all. God is up to the task; he turns my darkness into light. There was no way I could have pulled through without holding onto God's hand. His love is so deep, his mercy so strong, he sent people to me at the right time and place. Now I could be on my own, and I was happy to be by myself.

On Monday, May 2, 2016, I met with the doctor to remove the stitches. He saw that half of my body was terribly swollen and bruised, due to the leakage of blood drained into the wall of my abdomen from injured blood vessels where the shunt was placed. As my body rejected the shunt, blood drained into the abdomen tissue, causing it to show discoloration and tenderness of the skin. Bruises changes color over time. Initially, a bruise would be reddish, the color of blood under the skin. After a couple of days, the red cells begin to break down, and the bruise will darken to a blue or purplish color. About a week to ten days later, it will gradually fade back to its normal color. It has been over a year, and I can still see some purple color on my abdomen. My right breast was quite swollen and felt like a rock, very hard; I was in constant pain. Again, the doctor apologized.

I left the doctor's office and went to my appointment with my oncologist, Dr. Jacobson. He felt really bad for what I was going through, and he expressed how sorry he was. Another set of lab tests were done. After that, more extensive lab tests and examinations were performed every two weeks. About five weeks after the operation, I had a strong craving for white wine and champagne, even though I never drank alcohol; I talk to Dr. Jacobson about this. He said smiling "Champagne?" he thought it was funny.

I also wasn't sleeping at night, and during the day I might catch maybe two to three hours of sleep in whatever position I was in: lying down or sitting up. My television was never on because I could not tolerate the sound of voices. During my recovery from the operation, any little noise disturbed me; even the smallest noise sounded amplified. It was driving me crazy. Night and day I would think of the operation over and over. I could not get it out of my mind.

On my next visit to my oncologist, as much as I tried not to show my emotions, I cried a little while we discussed this. He told me I was experiencing post-traumatic stress disorder (PTSD). PTSD is triggered by a terrifying event that you experience and can cause flashbacks, nightmares, and severe anxiety as well as uncontrolled thoughts about the event. Now, besides dealing with my physical condition, I had to deal with a mental health condition! Prescriptions were called in for medication to help with my PTSD and my pain, along with a diuretic to help eliminate fluid. At last it was safe for me to slowly start taking diuretics. I was still exhausted from my liver not functioning. My eyes were very yellow, and my abdomen was badly extended. I got lots of questioning looks whenever I went out. I don't blame anyone for staring. After all, that was my appearance.

One day I ran into someone I knew at the grocery store. She gave me a strange look. "I'm having a health problem," I told her.

"Oh," she said. "I thought you were having a baby." That's the look I was getting from everyone: "Is she pregnant? At *her* age?" Taking the PTSD medication helped, but not entirely. I was still depressed. Were things ever going to change? Absolutely, yes!

7

DESPONDENT YET ELATED

I decided to have a talk with the doctor that did the procedure. Maybe that would help clear my head and lift my depression. I wanted him to know I had suffered tremendously. I also wanted to ask for his explanation of what had happened during the insertion of the shunt that had made him decide it was best I stay overnight. I wasn't unhappy that I had stayed; things would have been much worse if I had been at home, but I wanted to understand his thinking. I also wanted to tell him that considering the chance of rejection of the shunt and considering my particular condition with cancer, low platelets, and difficulty with clotting, another doctor should have been available to remove the shunt sooner. Nurses had not been able to reach this doctor. I thought it was neglect on his part, and I wanted to tell him so. I needed to hear the explanation from him. Maybe it would help me with the PTSD.

After making that decision, I called the physician's office a number times to try to get an appointment, but no one answered my call. I left three messages and received no reply to any of them. Three weeks later, while at the cancer center, I saw the doctor's secretary talking to someone in an office. She was leaving, but she immediately stepped back into the office the moment she saw me. I saw her peek out to see if I was still in the waiting area, and then she backed up again, out of sight. I got up and went to her. "Hello," I said. "I would like to make an appointment to see the doctor. I have left several messages asking for an appointment, but you have never returned my calls."

"What do you want to see him for?" she said.

"Regarding the procedure he did on me," I replied. "While I am here to see Dr. Jacobson, it would be a perfect time for me to see him."

"The doctor cannot see you today," she said. "Let me go to my office and check his calendar." With that, she left and returned a few minutes later saying I could see the doctor the next day at 9:30 a.m.

"Sounds good," I told her.

The following day I went back to the hospital to see the physician, and I was taken to a room to wait. When he came in, I heard him say to his secretary, "What is *she* doing here?"

A few minutes later, he came in to the room where I waited. He entered without greeting me, didn't even say hello. Instead, he said, "I thought the next time you saw me, you would walk in the other direction."

"Well, doctor," I said, "I am here today to get some answers. I'm hoping it will give me some peace, because ever since the operation, I have been reliving what happened over and over in my head."

"What is it you want to know?" he asked.

"When you were explaining the procedure to me, suggesting that it would be best for me, you said it was an outpatient procedure. What made you decide it was in my best interest to stay overnight? Don't get me wrong; I am glad you did. There's no telling what would have happened if I was at home when my body started rejecting the shunt. But I want to understand what happened."

"I never told you it was an outpatient procedure," the doctor said. "I don't know where you got that from."

"From you," I said. "You looked me in the eyes and said that to me."

"I never told you that," he said. I wasn't going to let his attitude intimidate me into silence.

"After the operation, why weren't you available, or why didn't you have another doctor available since you knew there was a chance of rejection?"

"I was available. I took the shunt out."

"You did remove the shunt, finally, after I bled profusely. You know of my condition with cancer, low platelets, and clotting problems. I suffered tremendously waiting and waiting for you. The nurses could not reach you; you were not answering your phone."

"No one was calling me," he said. "I can always be reached. Many times, these nurses have said they called, and I have checked my phone and found there were no calls. Don't listen to them."

"I heard them trying to reach you," I said. "I finally asked them to please call my oncologist, who, luckily, was in the building."

"What do you want from me?!" the doctor was shouting now. "Why are you here? Do you want an apology?" I ignored his question, and instead I showed him photographs I had taken of the bruises on the right side of my body.

"Perhaps it would not have been this bad if you had been available sooner," I said.

He chuckled, saying, "I don't want you think I'm laughing."

"Laugh all you want," I said. "I have suffered tremendously from your neglect."

"I can't believe you think I'm laughing!" he shouted. I had never seen a physician behave this way with a patient. I was frightened of him; he was so full of anger. I had thought my first oncologist, Dr. Sanders, was unpleasant, but this physician was far worse. "What do you want?" he shouted. "An apology? I apologized."

"You can keep your apology," I told him. I got up to leave, but overwhelmed from the ordeal, I didn't know which way to turn to get out of there. "How do I get out of here?" I said.

"You'll figure it out!" he shouted, walking past me out of the room. I heard him yell for his secretary, following it with, "Show this patient out!" I left the building near tears, feeling beaten and crushed, worse than I had felt before I went in. I could not believe the doctor had spoken to me in this manner. He had been verbally abusive to me. Here I was sick with a debilitating disease— cancer—and on top it I had liver failure. I was fighting for my life, and this doctor showed not a bit of empathy or compassion. He rejected everything I tried to discuss with him and was defensive before he even came in to see me. "He should be ashamed of what he did and of the inhuman way he spoke to me," I thought. "He is a disgrace to the medical profession." I consoled myself with the thought that at least he knew how I felt, and I was pleased with myself for confronting him.

A few days after that event, I started feeling better, physically at least. Emotionally, it was a different story. My depression continued, and speaking to that dreadful physician hadn't helped. His denials and outbursts were too much. I received no help from the conversation. To take my thoughts from that awful experience, and from my illness, I decided to turn to something I love, something extremely special to me: crafting jewelry. My intention in creating this line of jewelry is to show the beauty of the stones and found objects, such as sea glass, seashells, and sea beads, washed up on beaches. In two months, I created over two hundred pieces. It is always important to me that people wearing my jewelry feel beautiful and happy, but at this time these pieces were also my therapy blanket. People said I should sell the jewelry, but I wasn't ready. That jewelry was a part of me.

It took a long time to start letting the jewelry go, to give pieces to friends. Finally, I did, and it warmed my heart to do it. Eventually, I began selling my jewelry, with a portion of the proceeds going to the local chapter of the Leukemia and Lymphoma Society.

For the most part, the weight of my depression was finally over, but it checked in now and then. Sometimes I felt I was on top of Mount Everest, and other times I was struggling to get my footing on a rock to reach the top. Sometimes I was back in the operating room hearing the nurse yell, "What's wrong?!" and I was screaming, "I cannot breathe, I cannot breathe!" and other times I was excited for planning a trip to Hawaii, as well as thanking God for another great day.

In July 2016, my liver was starting to show improvement and the jaundice was starting to go away. Things were heading in the right direction. My distended abdomen was getting smaller, though it still felt tight and uncomfortable. I was extremely exhausted much of the time and had to rest a lot. I had been off chemo since the discovery of liver failure in February and was getting IV medication to boost my immune system. It was a daily uphill battle. Cancer is most unpredictable.

I started going back to church as much as possible, though I could only stay for Sunday bible study because of the exhaustion. My body missed my bed, and I had to lie down, but it was a good feeling to be with my church family. They were always happy to see me there, and they prayed for me daily. How awesome is that?

After being off chemotherapy for almost seven months, my IgM was rising. Dr. Jacobson suggested I give the chemo medication Imbrutinib another try. I had stopped this medication before because of bleeding, but I trusted him, and therefore I agreed to try it again. On October 10, 2016, I started the chemo, and after the third pill, the bleeding started. Still, I continued with the medication, hoping the bleeding would stop soon. It did not, so again I was taken off it. I thought to myself, "I'm off that chemo medication for good!" Even though my doctor thought highly of this medication, and it was the only FDA-approved chemo medication for WM, I was becoming afraid of it. But Dr.

Jacobson had what I could see was some good news. "The good thing about this chemo medication," Dr. Jacobson told me, "is that it keeps working on the cancer for a while after you stop taking it." And we could see those results: even without the chemo drug my IgM was still slowly going down.

At an appointment with Dr. Jacobson on October 26, he told me my liver was doing very well. The liver specialist he had consulted had told him in another year my liver would be functioning normally again. I wanted to get this liver condition behind me! He was saying it would take another year? I was disappointed, to say the least.

Dr. Jacobson suggested that because of the bleeding with the Imbrutinib he wanted me to start taking Revlimid again, even though one of its severe side effects is liver failure. I would be taking only one-quarter of the dosage, or one pill per week for one month, and he wanted me to start in two weeks. "I am not agreeing with it yet," I said to myself. I was thinking about my liver and having to wait another year for it to be normal. Taking Revlimid put me between a rock and a hard place: it helped my cancer, but there was a chance it could reactivate my liver failure. That's when I got the new idea. "Maybe I should concentrate on cleansing my liver," I thought.

I began educating myself about the types of plant and vegetables that were best for supporting liver function. I remembered my father's lessons about plants that are high in iron and that help with cleansing the blood. I read books on caring for a healthy liver, books like *The Liver Healing Diet*, by Michelle Lai, and *Nutrition for Health and Health Care*, by Ellie Whitney. After serious consideration, I decided to start eating mainly plant-based foods and organic fruits and vegetables and drinking liver-cleansing juices and smoothies. I wanted to give this a try for one month. I sent Dr. Jacobson an email stating that I would like to delay starting another set of chemo and told him I would like to focus on changing my diet instead. He gave his approval, and I started the new diet in November 2016.

8

A GREAT NEW BEGINNING

I was excited getting ready for this new transformation in taking care of my body. I would be focusing mainly on getting my liver back in top shape by depending heavily on organic plants, yet I knew this diet could help fight my cancer. A friend gave me a new power juicer, and I purchased a machine to make my smoothies. I went shopping for all organic vegetables and fruits and was ready to start my adventure of getting healthy.

On November 1, 2016, I started the new regimen. Every morning I would have a liver-cleansing juice consisting of red cabbage, red onion, radishes, celery, beets, apple, parsley, and carrot. These vegetables are powerful in cleansing the liver; they act as a detoxifier, helping purify the blood, eliminating toxins and waste, helping to keep bilirubin at a stable level, and helping to stimulate the overall function of the liver. Two hours later I had a fruit smoothie with berries, pineapple, banana, hemp seed, and protein powder, along with some soy or almond milk. Sometimes I would use water instead of milk, to cut back on the sugar content, as there is natural sugar in the fruits. I used all kinds of different fruits in my smoothies. My green smoothies were kale, parsley, sunflower sprouts, spinach, and green apples, with water and soy or almond milk. I drank two or three smoothies a day. For lunch, I would have a salad with broccoli, cabbage, Brussels sprouts, kale, chicory, and pumpkin seeds, with a vinaigrette dressing. My dinner consisted of baked sweet potatoes, fish, and some veggies.

After three weeks of eating these foods, I was feeling great in a way I hadn't felt in years. My energy level was higher, and my mind was clearer. My skin was smoother, my hair was thicker, and my immune system was stronger. I went in to see my oncologist for tests. Lab results gave good news: they showed my bilirubin was down half of a point. Things were looking up.

In December, I continued without chemotherapy. I just stayed on my organic regimen, and I felt super. Everyone was saying how healthy I looked as that challenging year came to an end. January 4, 2017, was another beautiful sunny day in Florida. I saw Dr. Jacobson, who was excited to tell me how much better my liver was doing. Lab tests showed my IgM count was going down without any chemo medication. I was doing great.

Words cannot describe how I felt hearing that. The best I can do is to say that leaving the cancer center that day, I felt like what a rose looks like when it first opens its petals to the sun. I was energized; I wanted to shout and tell the whole world how happy I was. Fresh juices and smoothies were going to be my new and healthy way of life, even if I had to go back to taking chemo. WM may be an incurable disease, but I discovered it can be effectively treated to allow for a good quality of life. I had always been a healthy eater, but the foods I ate before were filled with pesticides and other chemicals. I am much healthier now with what I am eating and drinking: fresh, organic fruits and vegetables in a mostly plant-based diet. Living with this disease has given me a new perspective on life; it empowers me. I have felt vibrant after starting this journey of organic plant-based foods, juices, and smoothies. I never fret about how much longer I have to live. Cancer is rarely on my mind. I have had the experience many times now in the waiting room at the cancer center where someone says, "You are not a patient, are you?" Those words remind me that, although I have cancer, it does not define me or run my world. I only live with it.

I dream now of traveling to beautiful, exotic places, to a world I've never imagined, to have a change of scenery, a new beginning. Cancer has helped me figure out what life is all about for me and where I fit into the equation. I am determined. I have an incredible inner depth that few are privy to and have the pleasure of knowing.

Since getting my cancer diagnosis, I had learned so much about myself, turning my focus from my next chemotherapy treatment to which veggie or fruit I might be juicing and what smoothie I might be having for my next meal. Learning a healthier way of living and to take care of my body more seriously has provided me with being the happiest I have ever been. It's a work in progress, but I have been improving my life even further by taking yoga classes and doing some meditation. I'm back to walking on the beach, too, and I'm loving it.

This disease led me down several paths, paths I thought were long gone from my mind, like having a romance; maybe I needed someone to hold my hand and say everything will be all right. With all that I was going through, I found myself having warm feelings for Ron, the kind and gentle man I had met at the hospital two years earlier. It took a while to recognize what was happening because I hadn't had these feelings for so long—more than twenty years. In that time, I had never had a desire for a companion. For as long as I could remember, one of my close friends would always say to me, "Elsie, you need a husband," and my reply to her was always, "I have no time or desire for a man." But here I was, filled with affection for Ron, this special and compassionate man. What was I to do? Should I tell him or keep my feelings to myself? To verbalize my feelings to him would be impossible. I was afraid I would be too nervous, that my words would come out like gibberish and their meaning would be lost. I decided to instead write him a letter and hand deliver it.

I love a new year. New year's give us a new beginning, and January seemed the perfect time to write a letter to Ron, confessing my feelings for him. In mid-January, after an appointment with Dr. Jacobson, I dashed over to Ron's office, said hello, and gave the letter to him. While he read it, I stood beside him, watching his facial expressions. He was smiling and seemed very pleased. When he finished reading the letter, he folded it, looked up at me, and gave me a smile. "This is very nice," he said. He tried to say more, but he failed miserably. Finally, he got the words out. "This is complicated," he said, "but something can be worked out."

"Call me," was all I told him.

A few weeks later, Ron called. My heart beat fast as I answered the phone. "Hello," I said.

"How are you?" Ron asked.

"I'm doing fine," I replied, but in truth I was feeling anxious, knowing he was calling in response to my letter.

After a moment, he began to speak, fumbling for his words, and then he spoke clearly and directly. "After considering your writing," he said, "I've decided it would be too complicated. My life is extremely complicated, and to add this would not be fair to anyone." His words came as a shock. Ron had shown signs of interest in me for such a long time. He continued. "I would like for us to stay the way we are, if that's okay with you."

"Oh, yes," my mouth said, while my mind said something else. I was stunned. Now I had another hurdle to get over. I pretended his words did not affect me. But they did. My heart was broken. After that, I sensed some distance between us. Ron treated me like a sibling. Yet I am not one to give up. I am waiting for the day his life will be less complicated and perhaps we will be more than good friends.

In the spring of 2017, I went back to work, giving the care that is so desperately needed. The work feels good, and I am so happy to be able to do it. Just a year ago I didn't think this would be possible so soon. What an awesome God we serve.

9

TIPS AND IDEAS

I never thought I would have cancer—and stage four blood cancer? It was not on my agenda, but I have faith in God to bring me through. Writing about my journey through cancer was certainly not on my agenda either. As I have said, I am an introverted and shy person. However, I have written this book with the hope that it will help others going through something like what I am going through. I share the following ideas and tips, as well, from what helped me through this experience.

1. Remember: cancer does not define you. You may find doctors that are good, doctors that are not so good, and doctors that are downright despicable. Keep looking, as you will find the right one for you. Don't be intimidated by all their medical credentials. They may know much more about your condition, but always remember that patients have rights. The doctors may be looking at lab results, but they cannot look deep into your soul at the way you are feeling. Try to educate yourself about your disease. Ask as many questions as you need to so you can have an understanding of your diagnosis and your treatment plan. You may be frightened; I know I was at the beginning of my cancer journey. But have courage and dig deeper

than you thought possible. Ultimately, you will find the strength and courage you need to go on, even when you've been dealt an unsteady hand.

2. In the very beginning, on my chemo days I always planned on having some kind of comfort food after my treatment—a hamburger and French fries, or KFC (a great treat for me). I figured I deserved to eat whatever I wanted after the unpleasant chemo treatment. That way, too, my mind was always on the treat, not the chemo.

3. I am not the most sociable person. I love my own company and was fine going to chemo appointments on my own. However, I know that many cancer patients prefer company when they get their chemo treatments; it helps them cope with the experience. If you are a cancer patient receiving chemo treatment, keep in mind that volunteers are available for just that purpose, if family or friends are not available. Ask your cancer center for a volunteer companion while having your treatment.

4. My experience with cancer treatment showed me the most compassionate nurses are in the chemo area of the cancer center. You are not just a number to them. They are more aware of your pain and anxiety than the doctors are, and they show empathy.

5. Some of your friends may associate your name with cancer; for instance, someone might say, "I spoke to my friend Elsie with cancer about going to the movie." I put a stop to that immediately. A lot of people think that showing cancer patients pity is comforting to them. I think that is not true. Pity is not comforting. I have said to a few people, "Please don't dig my grave yet."

6. For friends and family of someone with cancer: if you would like to help in any way, ask the patient what they need. Letting them tell you is more helpful than assuming you know what is right for them.

7. This tip came from a friend who believes in this strongly: everyone should have a "Go Bag" for medical emergencies and trips to the hospital or ER. This should be a large, brightly colored tote bag—easy to find. It should contain copies of medical information, doctors' information, insurance, and phone numbers of local friends and family, as well as a throw blanket, eye mask, ear plugs, moisturizer, extra eyeglasses, extra keys, a notebook and pens, and a good book to read.

EPILOGUE

No matter what, I know this: life is full of surprises, and I am ready for them all. About six years before my cancer diagnosis, I was taking care of a patient with dementia, a very sweet older lady. Her husband had died not too long before this, and I was one of three caregivers taking care of her around the clock in her home. As I do with all my patients, I gave her the best care, treating her with respect, dignity, compassion, and love. My shift was from 8:00 a.m. to 5:00 p.m., Monday through Friday. Along with her daughter, I accompanied her to all of her doctor appointments. I prepared three healthy meals for her daily. She was always clean and well-groomed.

One day one of the other caregivers said to me, "Elsie, why are you doing so much for her? She is not your mother." I was terribly sad and disappointed hearing those words from this caregiver. She was one of my mentors and the one who had gotten me into the medical profession in the first place.

I said, "She deserves nothing less."

Now, about six years after this patient's death, in my time of need and after going through several doctors who were professionals only by title, not by action, I have found one of the best, if not *the* best, oncologist, Dr. Jacobson. Dr. Jacobson has given and continues to give me the best care possible. He literally saved my life after my liver failure. To my amazement, not long ago I learned that Dr. Jacobson is the son-in-law of that patient I cared for six years ago, the woman with dementia. This discovery took my breath away. Remember: do unto others as you would have them do unto you.

Acknowledgments

I thank God for his guidance, mercy, and healing hands. His love is so deep and strong; his grace follows me daily.

Thanks to my family, who is helping me through this very difficult time. I love and appreciate you all.

I am thankful for receiving financial help from the Leukemia Lymphoma Society, which works with blood cancer research.

I am truly honored to say thanks to my wonderful oncologist, who God has put into my path to give me the medical care I so desperately needed and who saved my life on April 13, 2016—and who is still caring for me. You are my guiding angel and will never be forgotten. You have done a wonderful job helping me through my cancer experience.

Thanks to my church family, who prayed so very hard for me. I could never have pulled through without your prayers. Words cannot express how grateful I am.

Thanks to all my friends, who came to see me at the hospital, especially Ms. Burger, who saw me at my lowest point and was so scared for me.

Thanks to Tammi, who visited me so often at home with food and good conversation, even if I did not want to talk. She knew how to lift my spirits.

Thanks to Yasmin and Phara for visiting me at home, and for your words of encouragement.

Thanks to my friend Tina, who wrapped my abdomen with Chinese cabbage leaf. She was so sure it would take the fluid out! We are still laughing.

Thanks to Kim and Emily, who visited me at home with a very special lunch.

Thanks to everyone, even if your name if not mentioned, who has helped me on this journey,

These are the machines I used:
- For juicing: Cuisinart Juice Extractor and Jack La Lane Power Juicer
- For smoothies: Nutri Ninja Bowl Duo and Magic Bullet

Recipes

Liver-Cleansing Smoothie
1 cup red cabbage leaf
¼ red onion
2 radishes
1 red apple
1 cup parsley
½ cup carrot
1½ cups soy or almond milk

Blend until smooth.

Green Smoothie I
½ cup parsley
2 kale leaves
½ tightly packed cup spinach
1 green apple, core removed
2 T hemp seed
2 T hemp protein powder
1½ cups soy or almond milk

Blend until smooth.

Green Smoothie II
½ cup sliced celery
1 lemon, peeled
½ cup parsley
½ cup sunflower sprout
½ cup sliced cucumber
2 T protein powder
1 cup almond milk
1 cup frozen green grapes

Blend until smooth.

Banana Oatmeal Smoothie
1 large frozen banana
½ cup blueberries
¼ cup old-fashioned oatmeal
½ tsp pure vanilla extract
1 T hemp seed
1 T hemp protein powder
1½ cups almond or soy milk

Blend until smooth.

Carrots Beets Smoothie
1 cup sliced carrots
1 cup beets
1 red apple, core removed
1 cup red cabbage, chopped
½ frozen banana
1½ cups almond milk

Blend until smooth.

Berry Smoothie
½ cup frozen blueberries
½ cup frozen blackberries
4 frozen strawberries
½ cup raspberries
1 cup water
½ cup unsweetened apple juice

Blend until smooth.

Fruits Almond Smoothie
1 red or green apple, core removed
1 pear, core removed
½ cup pineapple slices, frozen
½ frozen banana
½ cup fresh or frozen mango chunks
1 kiwi, peeled
1 cup almonds

Blend until smooth.

Melon Smoothie
½ cup watermelon chunks, frozen
½ cup cantaloupe chunks, frozen
½ cup honeydew chunks, frozen
½ cup banana slices, frozen
½ cup sliced peeled carrots
1 cup soy or almond milk

Blend until smooth.

Apple Garden Juice
2 large carrots
2 beets

1 large red cabbage leaf
1 red apple, core removed
1 cucumber

Wash, prep, and juice all ingredients.

Leaf Apple Juice
1 tightly packed cup parsley
1 tightly packed cup spinach
1 large collard leaf
3 kale leaves
4 large romaine lettuce leaves
1 green apple, core removed

Wash, prep, and juice all ingredients.

Spinach Kiwi Juice
1 large cucumber
1 stalk celery
2 cups green grapes, frozen
2 tightly packed cups spinach
1 peach
1 kiwi, peeled

Wash, prep, and juice all ingredients.

Carrot Splash Juice
1½ cups peeled and sliced carrots
1 orange peel
1-inch piece fresh ginger root, peeled

Wash, prep, and juice all ingredients.

Fresh & Sweet Juice
1 carrot, peeled
3 beets, peeled
2 radishes
1 1-inch piece fresh ginger root peeled
1 red apple, core removed

Wash, prep, and juice all ingredients.

Green & Sparkle Juice
2 cucumbers
4 cabbage leaves
2 green apples, core removed
1 1-inch piece fresh ginger root, peeled
½ cup frozen pineapple chunks
½ cup frozen mango chunks

Wash, prep, and juice all ingredients.

Refresh Juice
2 cups fresh or frozen blueberries
1 large cucumber
½ cup fresh mint leaves
1 green apple, core removed
½ lemon peel

Wash, prep, and juice all ingredients.

Beets Pineapple Juice
1 large cucumber
2 beets, peeled
1 cup frozen pineapple chunks
1 1-inch piece fresh ginger root, peeled

Wash, prep, and juice all ingredients.

Berry Mint Juice
1 large cucumber
2 cups fresh or frozen strawberries
2 cups fresh or frozen raspberries
¼ cup fresh mint leaves

Wash, prep, and juice all ingredients.

Sweet & Refresh Juice
3 large carrots, peeled
1 large orange, peeled
1 cup pineapple chunks
1 cup fresh or frozen raspberries
1 1-inch piece fresh ginger root, peeled

Wash, prep, and juice all ingredients.

Fire Tonic Juice
My best friend Eli gave me this recipe. It helps me tremendously in avoiding colds and flu. I take 2 to 3 tablespoons daily for the first two weeks. Whenever I'm going to be out in a public area, I take 2 tablespoons before leaving home. I also use it as a salad dressing. The ingredients are easily found in health food stores. Bubbies' also makes an excellent spicy and hot horseradish.

5 bulbs garlic, peeled and sliced
1 yellow onion, peeled and sliced
1 2-inch piece fresh ginger root, peeled and sliced
1 T hot pepper flakes
¼ tsp cayenne pepper
Juice of 1 to 2 lemons
½ to 1 cup honey

1 5-ounce jar Bubbies' horseradish
2 quarts Bragg's apple cider vinegar

Slice all of the ingredients thin, so the vinegar can extract their essences. Add all of the ingredients, including the horseradish, to a large glass jar with a lid, and pour the vinegar over it. Stir just to combine. Place outside in the sun for two weeks, shaking the jar once daily. After two weeks, strain the contents using a stainless-steel strainer and then pour the liquid through a large piece of cotton cheesecloth. Pour this liquid into beautiful jars and store in a cool cupboard.

Scripture

Genesis 1:1-5

King James Version (KJV)

1 In the beginning, God created the heaven and the earth.

2 And the earth was without form and void, and darkness was upon the face of the deep. And the spirit of God moved upon the face of the waters.

3 And God said, let there be light: and there was light.

4 And God saw the light, that it was good: And God divided the light from the darkness.

5 And God called the light Day, and the darkness he called Night. And the evening and the morning were the first day.

INSPIRATIONAL NOTES

It was a special, warm feeling receiving a note or card from well-wishers. Below are a few.

Dear Elsie,

May a warm ray of sunshine find its way in everything you do today and pray that you are feeling better with each passing day. You are always in our prayers.

Dear Elsie,

How lovely! The colors of the bracelet you made me is so pretty. You add a little "wonderful" to everything that you do. Thanks for what you did for me, and thanks for being you! Keeping you in my prayers.

Elsie, may you take refuge in God's loving presents and His perfect strength pours into your today and tomorrow and after that. Hope you are gaining in physical strength. Love and prayers.

Dear Elsie,

Thank you so much for the beautiful bracelet; it is very pretty and extra special due to the make, it's so encouraging and uplifting to see you at service. I know you've been through such a difficult time, but your strength and endurance are amazing. Pease call us anytime you need something. We'd love to help. You remain in our prayers always.

Ms. Elsie,

Thank you so much for the beautiful bracelet! All the jewelry you made are lovely and unique for each person! You are such a blessing to us all. We miss seeing you, but know our germs are too dangerous for you. You are in our prayers always. Love

Elsie,

You are in my thoughts and prayers. Each time I pray for you I'm reminded that God who created you can put your world back together again. Please take good care and rest. May God grant you strength. We miss your lovely smile.

Elsie,

This card brings a boat load of love. Sure hope you are feeling better. We are about as usual, two old cripples holding each other up … Ha Ha … Sure, missing your sweet face at church, but know you need to be at home resting. Things will get better. Praying for God's healing.

Dear Elsie,

Praying the Lord will touch you with his gentle healing today. Praying for you. Love.

Elsie,

Know what my thoughts and prayers have in common? You are in all of them. We are so sorry to hear of your health setback. We miss you greatly. You are in our continual prayers. Let us know if we can help you in any way.

Much love.

Elsie,

Just a note to say hello, because you've been on my mind. Missing you. Love

Dear Elsie,

Wes are so sorry to hear of your resent setback involving medication; you are in our prayers asking God to take care of you and bless you with rapid recovery. We are so glad to hear you are now home from the hospital. It seems that you have had many obstacles to overcome, and your strength has been amazing and admired. You are a blessing to those around you. We pray that your medication and treatments will give you the ability to feel much better and be possible to be out again real soon. You are missed and kept in our prayers and thoughts always. Love

Dear Elsie,

When times are hard and hope seems dim, our hearts can always turned to him. So glad to hear you are improving! I know it takes a lot of rest and that by itself is frustrating ... be patient it will change. You may be shut in but not forgotten. If you need someone to grocery shop or pick up meds or others, please call me. Love and prayers.

Dear Elsie,

Laugh, smile, God knows your story. Thank him, Praise him, and give him the glory. We are so sorry to hear of your medication problems, and pray that it will soon be resolved. We miss seeing you at church and know that you miss being there. You are always in our prayers for comfort and full recovery. Love and hugs.

Dear Elsie,

You are in my frequent prayers for a speedy recovery. I hope you are feeling better soon and the day will soon be sunshine and flowers. All best wisher for you. We all miss you.

Sincerely.

Hi Elsie,

Thinking of you as I often do. You Lord are just in all your ways, and faithful in all your works; you are always near to all who call upon you. Take care and hope to see you soon. Love.

Dear Elsie,

You are in our prayers daily. I never got to know you the couple years I've been at the church but hoping this will change. Let us know if I can help in any way. We are praying for you. (Emily Richardson)

Dear Elsie,

With all my heart, I wish you a speedy recovery. You are an incredible person and deserve decades more of health and happiness. I feel assured that you will beat this. Wishing you warmth and comfort while you are sick. And once again I want to thank you for all you did taking care of my parents. I have always felt that your care and compassion toward my mother was instrumental in keeping her alive. I am forever grateful for that. Beth Corcoran

Dear Ms. Elsie,

I am sorry that you have cancer. I hope that you feel better soon. I am praying for you.

Dear Elsie,

*Thank you so much for the beautiful necklace. I love it!
It is exactly my style. That was so kind of you to think
of me. I think of you often, and I'm praying for you.
Every Sunday I look in your spot at church and say a
prayer for you. It is not the same without you around.
Please let us know if there is anything we can do for
you. We love you.*

Dear Ms. Elsie,

Thank you for the necklace. I love it! I'd love you to get better, and I miss seeing you at church. I will be praying for you. I love that the necklace was made by you. Hope you get better soon.

Love

Dear Ms. Elsie,

Thank you for the beautiful necklace. I love the pretty colors. I put it on as soon as I got it.

Love

Elsie,

This time in your life isn't easy, but you are walking through it with such a clear reflection of God's grace. Still there must be days that are harder than others, when you feel like this is more than you can handle. In those moments God's strength will be there to give you everything you need. Praying for you always. Much love.

Elsie,

Some people always seems to find a way to do something nice for someone; Elsie ... People like you! Thank you so much for my beautiful necklace. I love it!

My Dear Elsie,

I just want to let you know that you have a special place in my heart, and in my prayers. No matter what, God's light shines there for all to see. We send our love and prayers. Have a good day.

www.ingramcontent.com/pod-product-compliance
Lightning Source LLC
Chambersburg PA
CBHW030846180526
45163CB00004B/1471